Mainly Vegetarian, Mostly Vegan

A whole food diet that is good for you,
the planet, and your budget

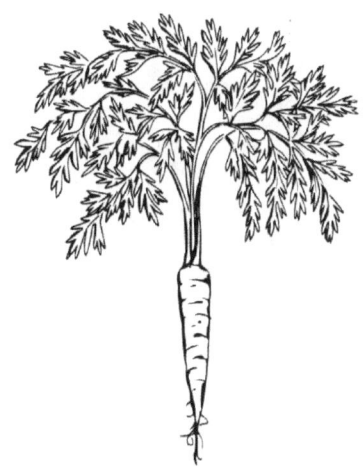

Michele Cornelius

DISCLOSURE

I am not an expert in nutrition and the information in this book is based on my personal opinion, my own experience, and research that I have done. I have included many of my sources at the end of this book so you can check them out for yourself.

I recommend specific products because sometimes the brand does make a difference in the quality and taste and I want the recipes to work out for you. I am not receiving any compensation from any recommendations in this book, and all recommendations are based solely on my opinion.

I do not assume responsibility or liability for any information included in this book or from any third party material that I recommend. Please do your own research before you make any changes to your diet. I am passing on what has worked for me, and hopefully this book will encourage you to make healthy changes in your own life.

"Nothing will benefit human health and increase the chances for survival of life on Earth as much as the evolution to a vegetarian diet." ~ ***Albert Einstein***

CONTENTS

Author's Note

Our diet is constantly evolving as new information filters in and we attempt to make good choices. It is inevitable that this book will require revisions, and I will do my best to issue a new version if it seems appropriate.

In 2012, I published **Definitely Vegetarian, Mostly Vegan** in e-book form and revised it a year later mainly to eliminate soy products. Once again, dietary changes have taken place. The largest required a title change since we moved to Southeast Alaska and have been tempted by abundant local salmon! Any time we are asked to dinner, salmon is on the menu. I am still conflicted about eating fish, and do feel strongly about not contributing to the large scale factory fishing industry that is so destructive to ocean life. We don't eat a lot of fish, and only fish that is locally caught in a sustainable manner. I am not including any recipes for fish and might give it up again, but not mentioning this as I put out a print version would seem disingenuous. Other changes include information on fermenting and probiotics, home wine making, and new recipes.   - *Michele, 3/2/2014*

INTRODUCTION

What if you could save money on food, have a cruelty free/environmentally conscientious diet, save time on food preparation, lose weight, and feel wonderfully healthy all at the same time? If this sounds good, keep reading. I have been eating a healthy mainly vegetarian and mostly vegan whole food diet for over 20 years and have developed menu plans and recipes that are easy, inexpensive, and good for you. I weigh less today than I did in my early 20's and keeping weight off is easy. Coupled with regular exercise, I am confident that anyone can be lean, fit and healthy by eating a mostly vegan diet of non-processed whole foods. With nearly 2/3 of American adults either overweight or obese (and other countries gaining ground), some drastic dietary changes are in order. We know fast food and processed food is bad for us, but get busy and think cooking at home takes too much time. We don't give enough thought to the consequences of our food choices on our health and to the planet. The answer is simple, and your meals can be delicious and satisfying. What have you got to lose?

While there is a section with some of my tried and true favorite recipes, this isn't just a cookbook. These days it is ridiculously easy to get a multitude of wonderful recipes with a quick internet search so traditional cookbooks are not as useful. This book will be valuable if you want to transition to a healthy diet and need more information to push you in the right direction. This book could be helpful if you want to lose weight. This book can be helpful if you want a complete solution with all the things you will need in your kitchen, what staples to have on hand, and menu plans to get you started. Even if you do want recipes, this book will give you basic recipes that are healthy, inexpensive and easy to prepare. A lot of vegan sites on the internet seem to be about finding substitutes for unhealthy comfort food, or about which brand of fake meat or cheese to use. This book takes a different approach.

The things I am about to say aren't news breaking; there is a lot of information on the internet, so do a search if you want more details or check out my reference list at the end of the book. I wanted to put it all together with my own personal spin in hope that my approach will resonate or provide the information in a valuable way. The American Cancer Society says that 1/3 of cancer deaths are linked to poor diet, being overweight, and physical inactivity. There is nothing more important than your health and diet plays a huge part.

1

MY STORY

When I was a child, I saw a sheep being butchered and it had a big effect on me. Our family was visiting my grandparents, and out on an evening walk we happened to pass by a ranch at the wrong time. I have always loved animals and the horribly violent scene made me think about what 'meat' really is and the idea of eating animals grew increasingly abhorrent to me (as it still is). My mother made me eat meat at family meals since she worried about getting enough protein, but I did what I could to avoid it. I slipped meat chunks into my napkin to toss in the trash later, and secretly fed some of it to our dog. I remember being made to remain at the table until I finished my liver and onions, and sitting there alone for hours. When I left home, I became a real vegetarian and haven't looked back. As more information filtered in, I became aware that the dairy industry is not humane and dairy products are not healthy for us or the environment so gave those up too. I've gone back and forth with it and occasionally cheat a bit with dairy and do eat eggs from local chickens or our pet ducks, but am committed to eating a mostly vegan diet because I know it is the best thing to do. My mother recently apologized for not supporting my youthful vegetarian impulses, and is now eating a lot of vegetarian meals herself! The tide continues to turn.

My partner in life is a guy who used to eat meat, but saw the error of his evil ways once I explained it to him. Gene was a chef when I met him and although he is now in a completely different line of work, he does a lot of the cooking since he enjoys it more than I do. Some of the recipes in the book are his creations, although getting him to specify exact amounts is challenging. We have many good recipes but for this book I am sticking with things that are easy, fast, healthy and inexpensive.

The truth is that I am at a stage in life where I don't want to spend much time or energy thinking about food or cooking. It is odd that someone who really doesn't like to cook is writing a book about it! I am not that into cooking, but we all have to eat and finding an easy, cheap and healthy way to accomplish this is a problem I have been trying to solve personally and it makes sense to share solutions I have come up with. I think our obsession with food is responsible for the increase in obesity and it would be better if we don't get into the 'foodie' recipes and fancy deserts that aren't good for us even if veganized. My goal is to share what I have learned in many years of researching and trying to perfect a healthy cruelty-free diet, and help others who are trying to do the same. If everyone went vegan, the world would be a better place.

I admit that I am not perfect and am in no position to judge anyone. I have gone back and forth about fish for years and occasionally cheat with dairy, although my convictions are firm. It is really hard to avoid plastic packaging and find things that aren't shipped for long distances. I don't want to spend all my time making things homemade or growing all my food. Modern life is complicated, and we do our best. Compromises are made, but we do what we can and any effort is better than none. I like to think that I keep on making small steps in the right direction and want to help you along that path too.

MOSTLY VEGAN DEFINED

I call my diet 'mostly vegan' because while I don't eat meat or dairy products, I do eat eggs if I trust the source and have recently included some locally caught fish. Some vegans get really uptight about it, and I know they would indignantly say I am not a vegan at all, but 'mostly' sort of covers that. Semi-pescitarian might work, but doesn't cover omitting dairy. Actually, it doesn't matter what label you use. What matters is that you make conscious decisions about what you will eat and what you will not eat based on your values and a respect for your health. I will not eat anything I can't kill, have a soft spot for all animals and can't tolerate cruelty of any kind so that narrows it down. I am trying to determine if fish suffer like animals, and that might change my mind about any fish consumption. It is important to me to be as healthy as possible and not consume anything that is bad for the environment, and for the most part animal products just aren't good.

We eat eggs that come from much loved pet ducks who are treated exceptionally well and given a healthy diet. We also eat eggs from local sources that are cruelty free. If I didn't have a good source for eggs, I would give them up although they are a good protein source and add variety to our diet. Egg protein has the right mix of essential amino acids needed for tissue building, high quality protein, 22 percent of the daily requirements of choline which is an essential nutrient for brain and memory function. Also, egg yolk contains vitamin D, carotene, calcium, iron, phosphorus, zinc, thiamin, b6, folate, b12, and pantothenic acid among other important nutrients. However, eggs bought from the regular supermarket are not a good option since the chickens were most likely raised under cruel and horrible conditions and fed antibiotics that are passed onto you. I will go into more details later, but the gist is that eggs are only OK to eat if you can see how the chickens (or ducks) are raised and know what they were fed.

Egg Substitutions - If you are (or want to be) a real vegan instead of mostly vegan, there are plenty of egg substitutes available. I would pass on packaged egg replacement in boxes with unpronounceable ingredients, but have heard through the vegan grapevine that Ener-g Egg Replacer Powder is less expensive and the best option. To substitute for one egg, add 1 ½ tsp. of Egg Replacer Powder to 3 Tbs of water and mix.

For more natural options, try the following: In sweet baked goods or deserts, a banana or ¼ cup of applesauce can be substituted for each egg called for. You could also substitute 2 Tbsp water + 1 Tbsp oil +2 tsp baking power for each egg, or ¼ cup chickpea flour and ¼ cup liquid. I have tried eliminating the eggs and adding more liquid in various recipes and sometimes it works and sometimes it doesn't. It depends on what you are trying to make.

3

WHY MOSTLY VEGAN IS BETTER

This could be preaching to the choir, but here are some reasons to give up eating all animal products (except maybe eggs as mentioned above) and most fish. Maybe you are on the fence and need a push, or maybe you cheat some and need motivation to stop. Once you have the information lodged in your brain, there is no going back without feeling guilty. At least that is how it works for me!

Animal products - The more I learn about the issues the easier it is to stick with the program. There is plenty of evidence that eating animal products of any kind is just bad. It is bad for the environment, it is cruel to the animals, and it is bad for our health.

The consumption of animal products contributes to all sorts of environmental problems such as global warming, pollution, water scarcity, land degradation, deforestation and loss of biodiversity. The worst part is the pollution; an average cow produces 60-140 pounds of mixed solid and liquid excrement which is usually flushed into a holding pond. This waste generates a lot of methane which is worse for the climate than carbon. Cows emit more greenhouse gases than cars, planes, and all other forms of transportation combined. Manure liquid can ooze from lagoons into the groundwater carrying nitrates, sulfates, chloride, and remnant antibiotics and dangerous bacteria such as E. coli, salmonella, and listeria. With huge factory farms, lots of material ends up in rivers and reservoirs altering and polluting the natural environment.

As for the cruelty issue, many people just don't think about it. In my mind, eating a cow is no different than eating a dog and slaughter house conditions are beyond horrible. Some people are so far removed from the source of their food that they just don't think of the shrink wrapped package they buy in the meat department as being a hunk of flesh.

You might think dairy products are different, and picture happy cows grazing in a field of flowers, coming inside in the evening to be milked. This rosy picture isn't the case for factory farms where most of the milk is produced. The 9 million cows living on dairy farms in the U.S. spend most of their lives in large barns or in feces-caked mud lots where disease is rampant. And you need calves to get milk, guess what happens to them? Some females are raised to become dairy cows, but most become veal. When the poor exhausted cows can no longer produce milk they are sent to slaughter house. Watch some PETA videos, if you can stomach it.

Even if the idea of killing or cruelly confining an animal for food or doesn't bother you, there are health issues associated with the consumption of dairy products. Most milk products come from cows fed high-protein soybean meal grown with pesticides, given growth hormones to increase production and injected with antibiotics to fight diseases induced by unhealthy conditions. All these chemicals are passed on to you. Even if you chose organic milk there are naturally-present hormones and milk, ice cream, cheese, yogurt and butter are full of fat. Eating all that fat makes you fat. It is a lot easier to lose weight when these items are off limits. I know plenty of overweight vegetarians, but no overweight vegans.

I have already covered some issues with eating eggs, but there is more to that story as well. While chickens don't need to be killed for the eggs, only females can make eggs so around 280 million male chicks per year are simply killed. Conditions at factory farms that produce eggs are just as horrible as those that produce meat or dairy products. Chickens are frequently packed into small cages and experience so much stress that they typically only produce eggs for 2 years at most compared to 15-20 years under natural conditions. They are used as egg-laying machines until they are worn out, then killed when they stop producing.

Fish - It is funny how often I am offered fish (or even chicken) after I tell someone that I am a vegetarian or vegan. Fish isn't a vegetable, but it is a gray area for some people. I have gone back and forth with fish over the years, and at times felt it was OK to eat only fish that I caught myself or wild fish in a sustainable fishery (if any exist). Again, it helps to get more information. There are lots of good reasons to stop eating fish from any source.

More than 40 percent of all fish consumed are now raised in aquafarms. The fish are cruelly confined in crowded net or mesh cages, and many suffer from parasitic infections and diseases. Most of the fish we prefer to eat (like salmon) need to eat other fish, and the aquaculture industry could end up depleting types of fish that are an essential food source for other species in the marine food chain. There are other issues with fish farms such as polluting natural waterways with excess antibiotic contaminated fish waste, the introduction of diseases to wild fish, and the possible escape of genetically modified fish which could decimate local fish populations.

Eating wild fish is not always a solution either. Besides the health danger from the high levels of mercury found in swordfish, mackerel, and tuna, there is the high fossil fuel consumption used by commercial fishing boats and the damage done to the ocean ecosystems.

With rising populations and the popularity of seafood, we have over-harvested the oceans and trashed our ocean ecosystems. Ninety percent of the large fish populations have been decimated in the last 50 years. The commercial fishing industry now uses massive ships that can stay out to sea for months with advanced electronic equipment to track fish, storing thousands of tons of fish on board in large freezers as they harvest more and more. Killing all those fish is bad enough, but all fishing methods catch and kill things other than their intended prey, like sharks, sea turtles, birds, seals, and whales. Scientists have found that nearly 1,000 marine mammals such as dolphins, whales, and porpoises die each day after being caught in fishing nets. Bottom trawlers scrape the ocean floor clean of life, and large nets scoop up anything in reach.

Living in accord with my ideals cannot involve eating food that is harmful to my health, the environment, or causes cruelty to any living species. Hopefully you agree with me that animal products and most commercial seafood are right out.

How do you get enough protein without animal products? This is a common question. In the past, it was thought that you needed to combine different forms of protein with each meal and have a specific amount of certain foods to get the right amino acid mix to get protein from a plant-based diet. Fortunately, this was later proved incorrect but the misconceptions linger. It really isn't that hard to get all the protein and nutrition you need. Eating a varied diet of vegetables, fruit, beans, grains, nuts, and seed will provide plenty of protein (and other nutrients) as long as you eat enough calories to maintain your proper weight. More protein isn't better, and too much protein can even increase the risk of osteoporosis and kidney disease.

The only thing that might be lacking is Vitamin B-12, and we take a supplement just in case since for the most part B-12 is found mainly in animal products. I have heard that B-12 was abundant in our soils but modern farming methods have destroyed it. In any case, it helps with many bodily functions like cell production, nervous system maintenance, red blood cell synthesis and DNA formation. Without it, you can end up with problems such as anaemia, neurological degeneration and digestion problems. Since it is so important, taking a supplement for it seems wise.

4

WHY UNPROCESSED
WHOLE FOOD IS BETTER

It is better for you, less expensive, and better for the planet to stick with whole foods, and I don't mean the market by that name although that is one place to get it. Whole food is unaltered food still in its natural state like vegetables, fruit, beans, seeds, nuts, and grains like quinoa, rice, oats or teff.

Grains should be whole grains that are not refined by removing the natural fiber and nutrients of the bran and germ. For example, whole wheat flour and brown rice are better than white flour and white rice. White flour and white rice are so common, but lack the nutrients in unrefined grain so why waste your money (and consume empty calories) when you could do so much better? There are some issues with whole wheat and we are now minimizing that in our diet (see the following chapter for more information). If we do eat wheat products, we make sure they are whole wheat and our rice is always brown rice or wild rice.

There is evidence that whole grains protect against heat disease, cancer, and diabetes and you have a better chance of getting vitamins, minerals, fiber, phytoestrogens, lignans, and antioxidants that are lost when the grains are refined. There are a lot of interesting whole grains to chose from, you can buy them in bulk, they keep for a long time, and preparation is as simple as boiling water. We eat primarily quinoa, brown rice, oats, and barley in soup but there others to try if you like variety. We just discovered teff, a very small seed sized grain renowned for its nutritional qualities. Teff is gluten free, has an excellent balance of amino acids, and is also high in protein, calcium and iron. I don't have any recipes for it at this point but it is worth looking into if you can get it.

If most of your food comes pre-made in little packages with a long list of ingredients that you don't recognize and can't even pronounce, you are not getting real food. Our processed and packaged food supply is full of artificial chemicals and additives for flavor, color, and a long shelf life. If you are going to buy something pre-made in a box or container, at least read the label and make sure you recognize the ingredients. You might change your mind when you see what is in it!

Another issue with processed food is the packaging. Purchasing your food in disposable packaging isn't the best way to go, even if the material is recyclable or recycled. You pay for the cost of that packaging, it takes energy and raw materials to make it, and so much trash ends up in a landfill instead of being recycled. Recycling isn't a get out of jail free card that absolves you of all responsibility. It is better than not recycling, but it is better yet to buy things in bulk without packaging and don't forget to bring your own reusable bags!

It seems clearly better to purchase whole foods in bulk and prepare them yourself. It might seem more difficult, but don't be swayed by that and end up eating chemical trash in plastic packaging. Cooking simple whole food isn't rocket science, and there are simple ways to get it done. Trust me, and keep reading!

5

CONTROVERSIAL ISSUES WITH SOY, GRAINS, AND GENETICALLY MODIFIED FOOD

It seems every time we turn around there is a study stating that something we are currently eating is bad in some way. This gets really frustrating, and it is hard to get good information since various sources are frequently in conflict. Studies are frequently funded by corporations who will profit from the results and biased information is the result. It is entirely possible that as I am writing this new information is coming to light that will render this inaccurate. It is always good to do your own research, but the following is my take on recent controversial issues with soy products, grain and genetically modified food.

Soy issues:

We eat small amounts of tempeh and miso because we like them, but there is some controversy about whether it is healthy to eat soy. After reading many articles about it, I came to the conclusion that eating organic fermented soy products in moderation is not harmful. The Okinawa Japanese are some of the longest living people in the world and they eat soy daily, but whole soy foods such as tofu, soymilk, and edamame as well as fermented soy in tamari and miso. The problem could be with the large quantity we eat, or all the processed products like soy protein isolates, soy protein concentrates, hydrolyzed soy protein, and partially hydrogenated soy oil. Also, it might sound like a conspiracy theory but it is possible that the meat industry contributed to the spread of rumors that soy is not healthy since it is viewed as a meat substitute. If you are going to eat soy products, make sure they are organic, and try not to eat too much of it. If you eat tempeh or tofu, it might be better to choose oat milk, coconut milk, almond milk or rice milk instead of soy milk. We used to eat a lot of tofu, too much, and have now substituted tempeh since it has less soy but still provides protein and delicious in many dishes.

Grain issues:

The bad news about grain (especially whole wheat) being unhealthy was the biggest shock. We had always been told that whole wheat and other grains were a good source of fiber and nutrients, and they form the base of that old food guide pyramid that recommends 6-11 servings! We know that quantities previously recommended are way too much, but to avoid bread and grain altogether is difficult. I have been doing some research on this, and the results have convinced me to seriously cut our whole wheat consumption and limit our intake of other grains.

A high wheat diet has been linked to obesity, digestive diseases, arthritis, diabetes, dementia, weaker bones and heart disease among other problems. On the Glycemic Index which compares the blood sugar effects of carbohydrates, both white bread and whole-wheat bread increased blood glucose more than sugar. In addition, one article explained that there is a connection between wheat and mental health problems since wheat inhibits production of serotonin which regulates mood and has some cognitive functions.

Also, if you are white, there is a good chance that you have some degree of an intolerance to the gluten found in wheat since 30% to 40% of those of European descent have issues. In addition, 1 in 133 people have celiac disease which is an intense form of wheat sensitivity that damages the small intestine and can lead to chronic diarrhea and cramping with impaired absorption of nutrients. A new report links the rise in gluten intolerance to GMOs, and I will go into that under the GMO section to follow.

While other grains are also suspect, it sounds like they are not as bad as modern wheat. Older forms of wheat such as spelt or kamut haven't undergone all of the modification as modern wheat. Decades of selective breeding and hybridization by the food industry to increase yield and optimizing characteristics of flour have created new proteins in wheat that the human body wasn't designed to handle. You should be safe eating quinoa, millet, amaranth, teff, and small amounts of brown rice which don't have the gluten and wheat proteins that trigger weight gain, inflammation and insulin resistance. We have switched to spelt flour, and plan to experiment with other flours such as teff flour.

Genetically modified food issues:

The final issue is with genetically modified food (GM food) or GMOs (genetically modified organisms) which refers to crop plants created using molecular biology techniques to enhance desired traits such as resistance to herbicides or insects. While these modifications can increase crop yields, there have been serious issues, serious enough that they have been banned in France and in some other European countries. The U.S. is in bed with Monsanto who creates the seeds and pesticides, so GM food is very widespread and has been declared safe despite evidence to the contrary. GMOs are in as much as 80% of conventionally processed food.

So why are GM crops so bad? It is bad for the environment since making changes in nature can have unintended consequences and do harm to other organisms. Plants cross pollinate, and genes can be transferred to non-target species. GM crops are also bad for our health. Studies have shown that GM corn causes organ damage in rats, mainly in the kidneys and liver, and also affects the heart, adrenal, spleen and blood cells. That is bad enough, but genetic modifications are also linked to an increase in allergens. Monsanto is powerful and will do everything they can to keep information from us, but it is likely that new health issues will emerge. I, for one, do not think it is worth taking a chance.

By law, organic products are not allowed to contain GM ingredients, but the crops cross pollinate. The biggest problem is with corn since they mix in the field, and around 1% of organic corn does contain GMOs. The only way to ensure that your corn products are not genetically modified is to buy blue corn, which is better in other ways as well. Blue corn has 20% more protein, and the blue color comes from a healthy antioxidant.

A recent report released in late 2013 links GMOs with gluten-related disorders. Although wheat has been hybridized for years it is not a GMO, nine GMO food crops are currently being grown commercially in the US : soy, corn, cotton (for oil), canola (for oil), sugar beets, zucchini, yellow squash, Hawaiian papaya and alfalfa. The problem seems to be that GMOs are modified to tolerate the weedkiller Roundup (Glyphosate) and the crops contain a high level of Glyphosate at harvest. Glophosate is a patented antibiotic that destroys beneficial gut bacteria, and an imbalance of gut bacteria is common in celiac disease and gluten intolerance. Corn and cotton are engineered to produce an insecticide called Bt-toxin that is designed to puncture holes in insect cells, but studies show it does the same in human cells which might be linked to leaky gut that it common with gluten intolerance.

It is hard to make decisions based on conflicting information being released, but always consider who is paying for the research and who will benefit from particular results. From all I have read, it does seem wise to limit consumption of soy, modern wheat, and completely eliminate GMOs. If you have concerns about it, do an internet search and see if you can find some truth in the conflicting information!

6

WHY ORGANIC IS BETTER

I've been there, staring at the slim pickings offered in the organic vegetable section of the supermarket, comparing a limp bunch of broccoli with brown spots priced three times higher than a crisp perfect looking bunch in the non-organic section. I understand the temptation to pick the non-organic option, especially if you are on a tight budget. Think about the real cost though and think about what really matters, like your health and the health of the environment.

Organic food is better for the environment. Organic crops are grown without the use of synthetic fertilizers, pesticides and herbicides. To do this, organic farms have found other ways to nourish crops like putting organic material back into the soil in a more sustainable system that nurtures a more diverse population of plants, insects and other animals. Organic farms use less energy and produce less extraneous waste such as packaging material for chemicals. Organic farms generate less carbon dioxide which is released in abundance in conventional farming by burning fossil fuels to manufacture, transport and spread nitrate fertilizers. Organic farms release no synthetic chemicals to harm the ecosystem or wildlife while in conventional farming chemical fertilizers and pesticides pollute drinking water, create enormous dead zones in the oceans, and release huge amounts of nitrous oxide which is a climate-destabilizing greenhouse gas. Pesticide use has been linked bee colony collapse disorder which is a huge problem world-wide since pollination is necessary for many important food crops.

Organic food is better for you. Studies have shown that organic produce contains more vitamins, cancer-fighting anti-oxidants, and important trace minerals. The most important reason to chose organic food is that over 400 chemical pesticides are used in conventional farming and residues remain on non-organic food even after washing. Pesticides are linked to asthma and cancer, and one class of pesticides (endocrine disruptors) may be responsible for early puberty and breast cancer. Some of the most hazardous pesticides that have been banned for use in the U.S. are still routinely used in other parts of the world that import fruit and vegetables to us (like Mexico and Peru), and testing for these is inadequately enforced.

Also, keep in mind that 'natural' doesn't mean the same thing as organic. Natural is over used on food labels to attract buyers looking for healthy choices, but it doesn't mean that pesticides weren't used in growing the food. Pick products labeled organic, and better yet grow your own vegetables without pesticides.

7

OBTAINING AFFORDABLE
HEALTHY FOOD

You can actually save money while eating organic healthy food. The downside is that it involves looking into different ways of obtaining your food and cooking it yourself. This might sound difficult if you are used to eating fast food and convenience food, but isn't as bad as it sounds and is worth it. I am not a foodie who likes to spend time in the kitchen, and the recipes in the book are easy and quick. I never spend more than a half hour making dinner, and usually more like 15 minutes. When I do spend more time, I make enough to last for a several days or put some aside in the freezer for future fast food. There are some wonderful restaurants that serve organic vegan food (and if I was rich, I would take advantage of this!), but it will cost you. Even a coffee shop habit adds up...You can save money by making coffee, tea and meals at home.

With more health consciousness in the general populations, it is getting easier to obtain healthy organic food from a variety of sources, even mainstream supermarkets. Most communities now have natural food stores with bulk sections. There are also increasingly more processed vegan food options in the natural food stores (vegan cheese, fake meat, boxes with packaged seasoning packets and vegan frozen dinners). These are expensive, and in most cases are not the most healthy choice. I do buy some commercially prepared products like tempeh and miso for the convenience but pass on all the rest. I am still struggling to find the perfect balance between quality, cost and convenience. Your line in the sand may be in a different place and like mine, might keep changing.

Dry Goods

Buying in bulk is cheaper, and it is way better for the environment to avoid all the plastic packaging. We bought lots of glass canisters from thrift stores, and keep them full of beans, peas, quinoa, brown rice, lentils, barley, popcorn, and oatmeal among other things. You can also use large glass jars for food storage, and might be able to get them for free from restaurants who buy certain foods (like artichoke hearts) in very large jars. We buy many items in 25 pound paper bags (beans, oatmeal, spelt flour, lentils, split peas, etc.). If you have a problem with mice or moisture, put the bags inside a metal garbage can with a lid. Also, if you are buying in large quantities make sure that you will use the food up before it spoils. We bought too much brown rice, for example, and ended up tossing it out since it became rancid.

The storage requirements of various bulk food items is more complex than I want to get into here, but there is a good website listed in the reference section at the end if you want to look into it. To sum it up, you should keep things in a sealed container to keep bugs and mice out, and most things keep longer in a dark cool place. Variations in temperature and humidity will affect how long things keep, but bulk items like beans, lentils, and popcorn keep for a very long time and you really don't need to worry about these going bad if you keep them dry. Brown rice will only keep 6 months, so buy that in smaller quantities.

The bulk section of your natural food store is good, but even that can be expensive. Look into food co-ops that allow you to purchase natural foods wholesale. In the U.S., consider going through companies like Azure Standard or United Natural Foods (it was formerly called Mountain People but is now a merger of other companies). With a minimum order (usually $500, you can order at wholesale prices and just need to meet the truck in a convenient place or pick it up from the shipping company. If you don't want to order $500 of food at once, you can go in with other people and form your own coop. There might already be a local coop that you can join. An alternative would be asking your local stores that carry natural foods since some will let you order through them in bulk although they do take a cut so the prices aren't as low.

Buying in bulk, you can save enough money to afford organic food. It takes some space for storage, but there is a secure feeling that comes from having a supply of food in case of emergency or shortages in this increasingly uncertain world. Be sure to do the math to make sure the price per pound is really lower. It usually is, and sometimes dramatically so!

Buying online - Shipping anything across the country certainly isn't green, but living in a small town in Alaska has some limitations and sometimes I can't find what I need or can get things way cheaper online than I can in our local stores. Bulk green tea is one item that we are getting online since our local natural food place is charging $27 a pound and I can get it for $11 online with free shipping. I rationalize that it would be have to be delivered to the store anyway. Not perfect, but it can save lots of money especially with the subscription discount and super saver shipping. I don't mean to sound like an advertisement for Amazon, but it is one of the ways I keep our food cost down. Sometimes the prices on Amazon are cheaper than our food coop.

Fruit and Vegetables

The best option is to grow your own produce, but it is challenging even in a perfect climate to grow enough to meet all your needs. There are plenty of other options to provide all of your produce or to supplement your garden.

Farmer's markets - While you can find organic produce in Safeway or Walmart these days, it is of course better to support small local farmers. Farmer's markets are an excellent place to shop, and they are becoming more common. Besides vegetables, some local farmer's markets also have bread or locally roasted coffee. There is something wonderful about supporting a local person instead of a big corporation, knowing that the product is wholesome and healthy, and being able to avoid plastic packaging. It is fun to meet the farmers, and the vegetables taste much better too!

Produce Coop - We have a produce coop that orders from the same place our local stores do, and are able to get wholesale prices by splitting cases of produce. It takes some work to figure out the accounting but once you have a system it can go smoothly and you can really save a lot for the effort.

If you get a good deal on cases or large quantities of produce, you can freeze, can, or use a cool root cellar to store the extras. In my experience, farmer's markets are too expensive to buy extra but with a produce coop this is a viable option.

Whatever source you use, look at the different options available and be flexible. Maybe you can pass on the organic corn and get less expensive organic cabbage instead, or maybe you can try something new. Eat what is in season and eat things that are grown in your area. For example, now that we live in Alaska, we are eating cool season vegetables that are grown here like broccoli, cabbage, carrots, and potatoes. We bought extra broccoli when it was in season and the prices were good, and blanched it and packed it away in our freezer for winter. We have a cool basement that keeps cabbage, apples, potatoes and onions fresh for months.

As a last resort, you can check the frozen section for organic fruit and vegetables. The produce is frozen quickly after harvest so has retained more of the nutrients but the plastic bags usually used for packaging is a big negative.

Grow your own - Vegetables, that is! This title comes from a sweet book I found at a thrift store for 50 cents on organic gardening. It was published in 1970, and has a cool hippie vibe with hand drawn illustrations...I love it! Simple, basic gardening information that is still relevant today. This book helped me understand the somewhat complicated stuff about plant nutrients (N, P, K) and how to add them to your soil with organic materials instead of buying commercial fertilizer. You don't need to know much to get started. There is a ton of info on vegetable gardening available on the internet, and it really isn't that hard to grow your own vegetables. Start slow, learn as you go. There is nothing like going out before dinner with a bowl to harvest your own crop.

I have grown vegetables all the places we have lived, and have at least been able to grow salad greens. The most challenging situation was in the Sierra mountains since the sun was blocked by big ponderosa pines and everywhere I tried to dig was solid rock. I ended up getting some large containers from the dump, filled them with purchased soil and put them in the spots with the most sun. I was able to grow some tomatoes, but mainly a steady supply of greens. My best gardens were in Sonoma County, California north of San Francisco. We were under redwood trees so had shade issues, but there was naturally good soil and a warmer climate. Now we are in coastal Alaska, but surprisingly our garden is doing very well. It is cool, but I can grow tomatoes in the greenhouse and broccoli, cabbage, potatoes, strawberries and lots of greens outside. Each location is different, and the trick is to go with what works best in your area. Ask around.

I like to keep it simple. I want fresh vegetables but don't want to work too hard for them or pay for soil amendments that come in horrid plastic bags. You need to start with good soil, and if your ground has been used as a garden before without adding nutrients or if it never has, you will need to add some. Our soil here was completely depleted and my first set of seedlings turned yellow and died! I should have done a soil test, but figured it out the hard way. We have been here a year now, and the compost I started when we arrived is ready to add to the soil (grass clippings, sea weed, moose droppings, coffee grounds, vegetable trimmings, etc.). I compost the easy way by just dumping material in a big pile, shoveling some dirt on it occasionally and turning it now and then. We have rain all summer so it keeps moist, but otherwise I would add some water. To get started while your are waiting for your compost to break down, you might want to buy some. In most places you can either have good compost delivered, or have them dump it in the back of your pickup truck like we did to haul home.

Picking up seed packets locally is the best way to go since usually they carry varieties that do well in your location. I grow 'arctic' varieties that have been bred to handle lower temps, for example. Some seeds can be planted straight in the ground (look at the package back for instructions) but I start of lot of them early in little pots in a warm sunny windowsill. After a season, you can save seeds from your own plants if you grow open pollinated non-hybrid plants. Buying plants instead of seeds makes it easier, but cost a lot more! If you spend too much, you might as well buy the vegetables from the farmer's market, which is a good option if you have the money and aren't into gardening.

I try to grow things that naturally do well in our climate, things that we like to eat, and things that are easy to preserve if we get too much. I am going to stash away potatoes for winter use and maybe freeze some things, but will otherwise just enjoy them when we have them. We frequently eat huge salads, and organic greens are sort of expensive but easy to grow. If nothing else, grow greens. We like spicy greens like mustards and arugula, but swiss chard and kale are also good in a salad or lightly steamed.

I could go on, but that would be best saved for a gardening book. Hopefully this gives you the gist of it. Growing your own vegetables is a completely worthy activity that saves your money, gives you something to do with your compostable garbage, gets you outside, provides exercise, and adds healthy organic vegetables to your diet. How perfect is that?

If you happen to live in a city, don't despair. Even a very small yard can produce vegetables as long as it gets some sun, and community gardens are springing up in unused urban spaces. Also, many vegetables do well in containers and can be grown on flat roof tops and on balconies. Even a simple pot in a windowsill can provide herbs and salad greens, and a supplemental LED grow light can be used if necessary.

Sprouting - You might consider growing your own sprouts, especially in the winter when it is too cold to grow greens in the garden. Sprouting can provide a continuous source of fresh, healthy, and inexpensive vegetables and it is easier than you might think. You need to buy seeds that are for sprouting, and of course organic is best. We use a mix that has alfalfa, broccoli, and radish. If you get into it, there are lots of types of seeds and beans to sprout, but we like the basic mix to put on sandwiches and salads. If you buy the seed in bulk, they can be very economical. There are all sorts of fancy sprouting systems available, but the fancy expensive ones are harder to clean and a mason jar with a screened lid works just fine. I only paid a few bucks for the lids, and used jars I already had.

Simply add 2 1/2 tablespoons of seeds to the jar, fill it with warm water and screw on the lid. After a few hours, drain and rinse them (right through the screen), then shake it upside down a bit so they aren't too soggy. Leave the jar inverted at an angle in a small bowl so it can drain and air will circulate in the jar. Rinse twice a day and shake the jar to get a lot of the water out and the seeds will begin to sprout. Once they have sprouted and grown to fill the jar, simply put the jar in the refrigerator. We have two jars, so we can keep one in the refrigerator for eating, and start a new one sprouting so we don't run out. Sprouts will keep for about a week in the refrigerator. Keep the seeds in a cool, dark storage area in a glass jar with an air-tight lid and they will keep for a year or more.

Free Food

Depending on where you live, there could be free food available. I am not talking about the freegan food taken from store dumpsters, although that works for some people. I am talking about wild food like mushrooms, greens and berries that can be collected in natural places. If you don't have natural land of your own, check into public park lands in your area. Some parks place restrictions on collecting, so be sure to check the regulations first and avoid places that might be poisoned by roadside emissions or industrial runoff. Always be completely positive about identifying any wild food before you eat it to prevent unintentional poisoning!

Wild Mushrooms - When we were living along the Northern California coast, we avidly studied wild mushrooms and collected many pounds of delicious mushrooms in the local forests to add to our diet. Fortunately, Southeast Alaska is also a mushroom hunter's paradise. Of course any discussion of wild mushrooms must be prefaced with caution since every year people die of poisoning from eating the wrong mushrooms. Once you know what to look for, there are plenty of delicious mushrooms that are very distinct from the poisonous ones and safe to eat, but be sure to study the mushroom guides carefully before eating any wild mushrooms or better yet, take a class or go foraging with an experienced mycologist. Some wild mushrooms must be cooked first, and many can be dried for storage. We have found oyster mushrooms, chanterelles, boletes, and many other wonderful mushrooms that are very expensive to buy in stores for free on our own property and on public state and national forests.

Wild Greens – If weeds grow abundantly in your area, it is likely that some of them are edible and can be used in salad or steamed as a vegetable. Dandelions have grown in all the different places we have lived, but I didn't try eating them until recently. The older leaves are bitter, but the young emerging leaves are good in salad. Nettles are also common in many wet places, but must be handled carefully and steamed to take away the sting before eating but are good as a spinach replacement in various dishes and make a healthy tea. In Alaska, we have fireweed growing everywhere, and the tender young shoots can be put in salads in the spring. Many wildflowers are also edible, like violets whose leaves have lots of vitamin C and taste delicious. Different things grow in different areas and it is impossible to cover it all, but you get the idea. It is worth researching the wild greens that grow in your area. I found a good book at our local library that was very helpful, but internet research might also pay off.

Seaweed - I tried to make pickles out of a bull kelp that we found on the beach and ended up tossing them out since the result was too rubbery, but there are other recipes to try and other varieties to experiment with. I haven't figured this out yet, but wanted to mention it since harvesting seaweed for food has good potential. If you live near the ocean (and have unpolluted water), it could be worth looking into. We love Japanese food and have purchased seaweed to use in miso soup, and getting it for free would be a plus.

8

MOSTLY VEGAN WHILE TRAVELING AND AT HOLIDAYS
✈

Being out of your normal routine can lead to cheating and exceptions to a healthy diet, but it doesn't have to! Here is how I handle it.

Traveling

I admit that is can be challenging sticking with a vegan diet while traveling, but it is getting easier to find healthy food in most places and isn't so bad if you plan ahead and have a strategy. There are some bleak areas in the U.S. near truck stops on major freeways that are limited to fast food or quick marts, and airports usually have a choice between junk food or expensive food so I usually prepare in advance and bring my own. There are various brands of bars (like Cliff bars) that can be purchased almost anywhere and are individually wrapped and easy to stow away in your backpack. I also bring a bag of raw almond and raisins which are healthy and travel well. If I have a lot of room (traveling by vehicle) I bring other things like carrot sticks, hummus, salsa and organic tortilla chips. When we are camping, I bring the snack food listed above and also things like oatmeal, bread, salad vegetables, canned (BPA free) organic soup, beans and chili. It is always good to bring some kind of food with you when you travel. There is nothing worse than being starving and faced with eating something that you don't think of as food. It also saves money since they charge lots more for everything in airports and quick marts.

In a pinch, there are usually nuts of some kind for a

snack in a lowly quick mart, and it won't kill you to eat pretzels. Sometimes you can find a little package of trail mix or some granola bars which aren't ideal, but will get you by. As for real meals, most restaurants will at least have a salad and even if it is iceberg lettuce served with white bread, you will survive. Steak houses always have green salad and plain potatoes, and you can usually get a sandwich shop to leave off the cheese and meat. Veggie black bean burritos without cheese or sour cream are my meal of choice while traveling, but make sure they don't cook the beans in lard. If you are more organized than I am, you can go online before your trip and research vegan restaurants and natural food stores in the area you will be traveling to.

I have not had a problem finding vegan food anywhere I have traveled, even in foreign countries. Vegans are common in England, I ate soup and bread in Ireland, plain pasta and salad in Italy, and beans with rice in Mexico. If you don't speak the language in the country you are traveling to, at least learn to say 'vegan' or 'no meat' or have it printed on a card you can show the wait person.

Situations can come up where you have no choice or the options are not practical and you might decide to relax your dietary rules temporarily. I would never eat meat, but on my last trip to California I ended up eating a grilled cheese sandwich since there was nothing else on the menu. It wasn't the end of the world, and I went right back to my normal diet. I did notice that it wasn't as good as I remember them to be! It tasted really greasy and heavy...tastes do change!

With some preparation, most of the time you will be able to stick to your vegan diet, but don't kick yourself if you blow it. Life is too short, and an occasional slip won't kill you.

Holidays

I don't know much about traditions in other countries, but in the U.S. our holidays are all about food. I want to get away from that, but end up feeling deprived if I don't get some Christmas candy or pumpkin pie at Thanksgiving. My grandmother was a small woman and thin, but a heavenly cook. She made the best flaky pie crust, and we always visited for Thanksgiving so I associate her in my memory with pumpkin pie. I still have the recipe card with her pumpkin pie recipe that she wrote out for me when I was old enough to make it for myself. I still follow her recipe every Thanksgiving, (with substitutions of oat milk, spelt flour, and coconut oil) and think of her. Food can be an emotional thing, and this is the time of year we are most likely to trip up. I do go astray from time to time but try not to kick myself for it. Life is short, and perfection in our diet or anything else would render us harsh and inflexible. Just try to get back on track after the holidays are over!

For Thanksgiving, we usually have tofu turkey (either Tofurkey or our own homemade concoction), roasted vegetables, wild rice, cranberries and pumpkin pie. We have treats like special liquors at Christmas, and things made with dark chocolate. After eating healthy food for a while your tastes change, and the cookies made with white flour and frosting don't even look good. Don't send them to me for Christmas, since I will toss them out! I still crave chocolate though, and make dark chocolate truffles. But only at Christmas.

"Going meat-free can make a huge difference. Studies show that vegetarians are, on average, 10 to 20 pounds lighter than meat-eaters and that a vegetarian diet reduces our risk of heart disease by 40 percent and adds seven or more years to our lifespan." - **Ingrid Newkirk**

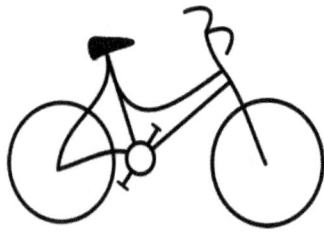

9

LOSING WEIGHT AND GETTING FIT
⸙

The saying "eat to live, don't live to eat" is so true. But how can we develop a healthy relationship with food? Being healthy should be a priority, since without that you have nothing. It is complicated though, and people are too busy, unhappy and distracted. Food has become a reward and a comfort instead of body fuel. Not that healthy food can't be delicious, but it is better to think about it in a different way. The key to getting back on track is basic: eat whole natural foods when you are hungry. That sounds simple enough, but many of us have problems with it.

When I was younger and working, I definitely had an emotional relationship with food. Spending most my day slaving away at a desk, lunch was a highlight. Then were the treats in the break room, the candy hidden in my desk drawer to get me through an unpleasant day. I ate at scheduled times, not because of hunger.

We lived in the wine country of California years ago, and got into the foodie things like good bread, wine, cooking fancy meals with expensive ingredients. We were too cheap to go out to eat much, but there was some of that too. We thought too much about what to have for dinner, and spent too much time preparing it. We have always exercised a lot and have never been into junk food, but you can get fat with a vegetarian organic diet that includes cheese, butter, chocolate and pasta. We didn't have a problem with weight until our 30's...It gets much harder with age, unless you inherited one of those enviable metabolisms that keep you thin no matter what. We found solutions though, and are much better for it.

Eat when you are hungry. Don't eat because it is 12:00, or 6:00. When you wait for hunger, it helps get things back in balance. You will crave things your body needs, and it takes the 'emotional' element out of the equation. Don't wait until you are overly starving though, have snacks like raw almonds, apples, carrots, or air popped popcorn that you can grab. Have the ingredients on hand for easy and quick meals.

Eat slowly, and eat less. If you eat too fast, your stomach doesn't register that it is full until it is too late and you have over eaten. Eating too much at once makes you feel tired and sluggish as your body tries to digest it all.

Think of food as fuel. Eat healthy, nutritious whole foods. Don't have junk or processed food in the house. Stock oatmeal, fruit, beans, brown rice, quinoa, raw nuts, and seeds. Drink water or green tea instead of soda.

Don't obsess about food. Keep meals simple, and try not to use food as a reward, celebration or consolation.

Don't go out to eat often and if you do, make good choices. Most menus offer salads. Japanese food is often a good choice, things like vegetarian sushi and miso soup. A typical entree is too large for one person so split it with a friend or take half home for later.

It doesn't need to be too harsh, have a glass of wine with dinner or a beer with lunch. Have a small handful of dark chocolate chips if you feel like something sweet. If you generally make good choices, and keep things in moderation, it will be fine.

The good news is that if you can stick with it and develop good habits, your tastes eventually change. Junk food doesn't look or sound good anymore; it is too salty and seems gross. I tend to crave fruit, nuts or a healthy salad. I am over 50 now, and am still a size 8. I have a lot of energy, exercise at least an hour a day and have no health problems. I have always wanted to be thinner, but part of that is the ingrained Hollywood view of perfection and not the ideal goal of being healthy. If you are overweight, don't put off making steps towards change. It isn't easy, but you can develop healthy habits.

Exercise – This book is about food, but that is only part of the equation. To be healthy and maintain a normal weight, you need to incorporate exercise into your daily routine. Studies show that exercise improves cardiovascular health, lowers blood pressure, and improves metabolism and levels of cholesterol and trigycerides. It reduces diabetes risk and the risk of certain cancers. Exercise makes you feel good physically and mentally, and the longer you keep it up, the better it feels. Once you are in good shape, working out isn't difficult at all. The hard part is developing the habit.

One secret is to find something that you enjoy doing. I love being outside and time flies by when I am hiking, biking or snow shoeing. If you exercise outdoors like I do, it is good to have a backup plan for when the weather is bad although rain and snow gear is always an option.

It also helps to get exercise doing normal things throughout your day, like climbing up stairs. Our current house is on three levels, and going up and down the stairs helps keep us fit. Doing chores and yard work yourself is good. Rake leaves, shovel snow, dig in the garden. Walk around town instead of driving, and better yet bicycle to town. There are a lot of ways to get exercise without even trying in your normal routine.

In addition, it is good to fit in a half hour a day for a more intense workout. It can even be 15 minutes in the morning and 15 minutes in the evening. You don't need a gym membership or fancy equipment, and a small mat or rug in your living room will work fine. Current info shows that interval training is better than prolonged sessions, and it might even protect your heart to have short burst of exertion followed by periods of rest. I like to do a type of circuit training with a variety of exercises that are repeated. The high-intensity phase should be strenuous enough to get you breathing heavy, followed by a recovery period. I like to do jumping jacks to get my heart rate up, then lift two 6 lb weights until my arms are tired, then do squats, then burpies, then mountain climbers, then push-ups, then lunges, etc. After resting, I do the circuit again or do it at another time during the day. Yoga is also highly recommended for relaxation and flexibility.

Studies have shown that sitting at a computer for hours at a time is not good for us, even if we get exercise later in the day. Standing desks are good, or you could get up every hour or so and do some jumping jacks or mountain climbers. Set an alarm if you tend to forget! You might be embarrassed doing this at work, but it will improve your concentration and your health. Even getting up to walk around will help.

Swim, walk, run, hike, paddle, peddle or whatever sounds good to you, but keep moving!

10

ALTERNATIVE COOKING METHODS
✿

Being an environmentalist on a budget, I am interested in exploring alternative ways of cooking that don't involve using the typical gas or electric stove. I realize some people will not be interested in this, so if you aren't just skip this section.

In the winter, we frequently cook on the wood stove since it is going 24-7 to keep us warm and is a free heat source since we have plenty of downed wood. It makes sense to heat water using a kettle on the wood stove, and it is also perfect for cooking beans, grains, soup and various other things that would otherwise be cooked on a burner. There are ovens for wood stoves, but we don't have one and my attempts at using modified camping ovens on the top of our stove failed miserably. I have had great success making cornbread in a cast-iron skillet like a big pancake. We have metal diffusers that stack and are used under the pot to control the temperature when the fire is too hot, and sometimes it is necessary to add more wood or open the damper to make the fire hotter. Generally I like to use it like a slow cooker for things like soup or beans that aren't particular about temperature and just check them now and then when I think about it and it all works out fine.

In the summer, we frequently use a solar oven for beans and grains. Solar ovens can even work on a sunny day in winter since it isn't dependent on warm outside temperatures, but in Alaska the low angle of the winter sun makes this almost impossible. There are different brands available and I chose the Global Sun Oven because of portability. You can build one for much less, and even a cardboard box with foil will work but it takes a bit more engineering to get high temperatures (like 400 degrees) which is useful for baking bread. A durable homemade solar oven out of wood, aluminum and glass would be larger and heavier, and would take effort to build. The sun oven we have folds up into a small case and has a handle which makes it easy to store in the winter and take with us on camping trips.

You can cook almost anything in a solar oven, although I usually use it mainly for beans, rice, spelt, and various grains. I like the fact that nothing seems to burn even at high temperatures. There is a thermometer so you can see how hot it is getting, and you can make it cooler by tilting it away from the sun. I don't tend to time my cooking, and just check on it when I remember, but it always seems to work out. Once I left some muffins in there for and hour and a half, and they were still edible. Probably because the sun moves and if you don't adjust the oven every now and then it starts cooling off.

The best use of the oven is for cooking beans since they take so long to cook on the stove. You just put 1 cup of dried beans and 2 cups or more of water in a casserole dish with a clear glass lid and stick them in the solar oven facing the sun. Soaking first makes them cook faster, but I don't usually bother. Adjust the oven a few times as the sun moves, and they should be done in 4 hours but it is fine to leave them in longer. You can make a big batch and put serving sizes in the freezer for 'fast food'.

With most electricity coming from nasty coal and prices rising higher, why not try cooking with free energy from the sun or your wood stove? It is easier than you think.

11

MEAT AND CHEESE SUBSTITUTES

👀

I didn't like the taste or idea of meat before I became mostly vegan, so having fake sausage, ribs, or hot dogs sounds unappealing. Veggie burgers are yummy, and often the only vegetarian choice on a menu but not because they taste just like a hamburger - it is the bun and fixings. There are lots of options in the natural food stores, but they break my non-processed food rule, the ingredients are suspect, and they are expensive. Substitutes have been helpful to those trying to make the transition to a vegan diet but be especially wary of item like seitan that is high in gluten.

We occasionally buy a tofu turkey for Thanksgiving, but have also successfully made our own. Tempeh is sort of like a meat substitute, and is our current favorite. It can be sliced and browned with soy or barbeque sauce, it can be crumbled and added to many dishes for extra protein and flavor.

One of the hardest things for me to give up was cheese since I have a thing for pizza, and I spent some effort looking for a substitute but was not impressed with either store bought versions (pricey plastic wrapped tasteless concoctions with unknown elements) or recipes I found online. Some recipes came out looking and tasting like big blocks of Velveeta (gross American cheese) and were not even good in sandwiches. Many recipes require ingredients that were hard to find and/or expensive, and took too long to make so I eventually gave up on the idea. Nutritional yeast can add a cheese-like taste to things, is easy to find in the bulk section, and is good for you. We use it in several of our recipes and also add it to popcorn.

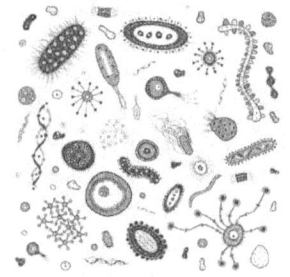

12
FERMENTATION AND PROBIOTICS

Although I spend many years nursing a Kombucha culture in sweetened tea and drinking the vinegar like liquid daily because it was supposed to be healthy, I didn't fully understand why and eventually killed off my culture by leaving it in a cold house. Reading Michael Pollan's book *Cooked* (skip the meat parts!) led me to research fermentation, and now I have several mason jars of vegetables on the counter fermenting away, as well as a jar of water kefir. I might even order another Kombucha scopy! I am convinced that the probiotics these provide could be healthy although I haven't been able to physically tell the difference. Besides the possibility of probiotics, fermenting is a great way to preserve extra vegetables and the water kefir makes a tasty beverage.

I had previously dismissed vegetable fermentation since sauerkraut always seemed horrible, a grayish mass of sour cabbage paired with disgusting meat. Now that I am preparing my own with carrots, ginger, and my own favorite seasonings it is an entirely different experience. The vegetables remain crisp and colorful, and the sour tang is wonderful. I have barely scratched the surface of the different vegetable combinations that can be fermented, but it doesn't need to have cabbage or taste like sauerkraut. Onions, garlic, broccoli and red peppers are very good fermented with a little cumin, and when I have tomatoes again I will try a fermented salsa.

You might be able to find fermented food in the refrigerator section of your health food store, but they will be expensive. Most supermarket versions of fermented food are overly processed with high heat which destroys the nutrients and the probiotics. Luckily, it isn't hard to make it yourself.

Why Fermented Foods are Healthy

Fermented foods undergo a process of lactofermentation, where natural bacteria feed on the sugar and starch in the vegetables creating lactic acid. The process preserve the food, and breaks down the food into a more digestible form as well as creating probiotics that are said to improve digestion, promote the growth of healthy bowel flora, and protect against diseases of the digestive tract. Having the proper balance of gut bacteria and enough digestive enzymes help you absorb more of the nutrients in the foods you eat. Some scientists say up to 80% of our immune systems are contained within our gut, so having a good balance of probiotics can help heal infections and stave of illness. I have also read that probiotics can benefit everything from allergies, dental cavities, weight loss and protecting against colon cancer. I don't know if all the claims are true, but it is worth eating fermented food even if only some of them are. One source recommended eating ¼ cup of fermented vegetables a day, and that is my current goal.

An internet search will give you plenty of recipes if you are interested in trying it, and there are a variety of containers that would work ranging from expensive crocks to mason jars with something to weigh down the vegetables. You don't want the vegetables to be exposed to oxygen or mold will develop. Some articles say that you can just remove the mold, but others say once you can see it, there are tendrils extending down into the jar and it is better to toss it out. Also, if it starts to smell bad, you probably have something undesirable growing in your culture.

After reading lots of articles, I am convinced that it is best to use an airlock. They sell expensive setups for this purpose, but the cheapest way to get started is with a cap for a wide mouth mason jar that you probably already have or can find at a thrift store. I purchased a lid called reCAP, and the hole in the top perfectly fits a #6 rubber stopper that is pre-drilled for an airlock. The lid, stopper, and airlock can all be found on online, and none of these are very expensive. I have had no mold at all in my fermentation experiments using the airlock. When I tried weighting the vegetables down in the jar, it was difficult to keep it from floating up around the edges.

I won't give an exact recipe because I do it differently every time, but basically you chop up some vegetables in a big bowl and sprinkle them with salt. Then you pack them into a wide mouth mason jar, pressing them down with the bottom of a glass to pack them in. It takes more than you would expect since they pack down quite a bit!

For one jar, you might try a head of cabbage, a large carrot, and grated ginger with one tablespoon of non-iodized sea salt (salt helps with preservation). Another combination we really like is broccoli, onion, garlic, freshly grated turmeric, and cumin. As you press it down, the salt pulls out the liquid in the vegetables, and the level keeps rising. Keep smashing it down with the bottom of the glass now and then, and leave it on the counter overnight. In the morning, if the juice hasn't covered the top of the vegetables, add some water and screw on the top with the airlock. Some sites recommended testing it every week to taste but apparently the fermentation is the most healthy for you after four weeks when the conversion process is more advanced. To stop the fermentation, simply remove the airlock, cap the top and store it in the refrigerator. It will keep for months, but we haven't tested this since we end up eating it within a few weeks.

Water kefir is another source of probiotics, and is fairly easy to maintain. Water kefir (also called Tibicos among other things) is a culture of bacteria and yeasts, and the microbes present act in symbiosis to maintain a stable culture if kept in sugary liquids. They feed off the sugar producing lactic acid, alcohol, and carbon dioxide which carbonates the water. Supposedly, water kefir is loaded with valuable enzymes, easily digestible sugars, beneficial acids, vitamins and mineral and supplies your body with billions of healthy bacteria and yeast strains.

I purchased my water kefir online, and received a little zip lock bag with some semi-moist translucent lumps. I followed the instructions to get them started, and now add one teaspoon of molasses and 1/3 cup of organic sugar to a jar with ½ cup of kefir grains every other day after straining out the finished liquid. I store it in the refrigerator to stop the fermentation, although some people leave it out longer to create more fizz. You can add fruit or flavoring, but it tastes fine to me unadulterated. We dump the kefir water in our morning smoothie which works well and adds some sweetener.

13

THE BASICS: EQUIPMENT AND STAPLES TO KEEP ON HAND

Equipment

I like to be as minimal as possible, but if you are going to cook healthy food at home you will need some decent kitchen equipment. You might think one pot will do, but what if you have two things cooking on the stove at the same time, or have leftovers in a pot in the refrigerator and want to cook something different? I like to store things in the pot if they are going to be reheated since it is easier than washing out another storage container. I am not a fan of having lots specialized kitchen equipment when something common will work or owning things that are rarely used, but having what you need makes life easier.

All of our kitchen gear was purchased at thrift stores and garage sales, and I frequently see used stainless steel pots. They might need a bit of cleaning up, but it is better to get good quality, expensive brands used than buy cheap brands new. Good quality stainless steel or cast iron pans will last your lifetime and then some.

Since we are talking about being healthy here, don't take chances with Teflon or nonstick cookware which has been found to release toxic gases when heated to certain temperatures. I don't even use a microwave since I have read some bad things about it, especially in regards to plastic containers. You can make your own decisions, but I advocate cooking, baking and storing with stainless steel, ceramic, cast iron or glass.

The experts keep changing their mind about what is harmful and what is not, but plastic is suspect, especially those with BPA, which is in polycarbonate plastic typically marked with a number 7 on the bottom. It has been known since 1936 that BPA mimics estrogens and is linked to increased breast and prostate cancer, altered menstrual cycles and diabetes in mice. Studies show that it leaches from plastics and resins when they are exposed to hard use or high temperatures (such as microwaves or dishwashers). The U.S. Centers for Disease Control found traces of BPA in nearly all urine samples it collected in 2004 as part of a study to determine the prevalence of chemicals in the human body. While experts are split on the potential health hazards to humans and some say that our bodies flush it out, I don't think it is worth the risk. Some studies are funded by the same chemical companies that produce harmful substances and can't be trusted.

We might not know the full ramifications of all the chemicals we are exposed to in modern life for years to come, and then it will be too late. Cancer rates are increasing, and it seems clear that it is all the chemicals we are exposed to. I am not very social, and still know five women who have had breast cancer and two men with prostate cancer. Under the circumstances, it seems reasonable to avoid using plastic in contact with our food. No plastic spatulas, plastic storage containers, plastic bowls, plastic water bottles, plastic cups (or canned food with BPA liners).

The following is a list of things I recommend having in your kitchen. This isn't a minimalist kitchen and it can be done with less, but these are things that make cooking your meals at home easier. If you are cooking for 1 person and or don't have other people over for dinner, your needs may vary but this is my complete list.

Equipment list:

- 1 large stainless steel pot for boiling pasta or steaming vegetables
- 1 large ceramic soup pot (This makes life easier because you can cook with it on the stove and then stick it in the oven. Otherwise you might have to transfer the contents into a different casserole dish to bake which makes for more dish washing.)
- 1 medium pot
- 2 small sauce pans
- 2 cast iron skillets
- 1 strainer
- 1 stainless steel collapsible steaming basket
- 1 cookie sheet
- 1 Pyrex-like baking dish
- 1 Pyrex-like glass casserole dish
- 1 glass liquid measuring cup (2 cup)
- 1 set of stainless steel measuring cups
- 1 set measuring spoons
- 2 wooden spoons
- 1 large mixing bowl and 1 smaller bowl
- 1 stainless steel spatula
- 1 large serving spoon (to scoop soup out with)
- 1 silicone rolling mat and rolling pin for tortillas
- 1 stainless steel tea kettle
- A set of glass storage containers with lids for leftovers
- Lots of glass canisters and jars for storage of bulk items
- Blender
- Toaster
- Air-popped Popcorn Popper
- Soy milk maker (for making oat milk)
- Wooden cutting board (one side for onions or garlic, one side for bread)
- Set of kitchen knives that includes a bread cutting knife, 2 paring knives, 1 chopping knife

Staples to keep on hand:

We buy things in bulk whenever possible since it saves money and avoids packaging.

Bulk items-
Spelt flour
Walnuts
Sunflower seeds
Raw almonds
Quinoa
Raisins
Seeds for sprouts
Lentils
Split peas
Black beans
Teff
Oatmeal
Steal Cut Oats
Flax seeds
Brown rice
Barley
Popcorn
Garbanzo beans
Nutritional yeast
Coffee and tea
Spices – chili powder, garlic powder, onion powder, cumin, season salt, peppercorns, oregano, cayenne pepper, curry spice
Vegetable bouillon (cubes or equivalent)
Baking powder, baking soda

Sweeteners -
Gallon jug of unsulphured molasses

Honey – Local is best since it is unlikely to be processed like supermarket honey. Some honey has the pollen and nutrients removed, and has added sugar.

A note about sweeteners - All the sugar options in the natural food stores these days can be confusing – powders, syrups and liquids all claiming to be healthier and more environmentally-friendly. Some of these are much more expensive, and after researching the options we have decided to go with molasses or honey when possible since they still contains some nutrients. Sugar is not healthy in any form, and isn't a significant source of vitamins or minerals. We keep some granulated organic sugar around for when the flavor of molasses or honey would not work. We pick the cheapest organic option, and try to use as little as possible.

Canned goods (BPA free)-
Beans, tomatoes, pumpkin

Misc. glass jars –
Soy sauce, olive oil, salsa, organic spaghetti sauce, rice wine vinegar, mustard, tahini

Coconut oil - Coconut oil has become our butter replacement. With a sprinkling of salt, it is good spread on bread and it works well in recipes calling for butter. I am also making natural deodorant and hand lotion from coconut oil. It is very useful to keep around.

Perishable goods for storing in a dry, cool place -
Garlic, onions, carrots, potatoes, apples

Frozen – Ginger, turmeric, berries, bananas

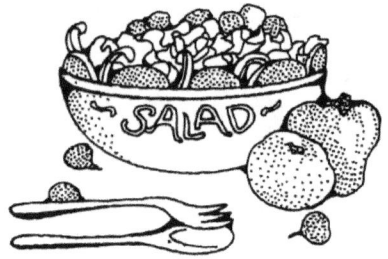

14

MEAL PLANS
🍴

The goal is to eat a healthy, inexpensive diet with minimal time spent in preparation and planning. Some people really love to cook and it becomes a hobby; I am not one of those people. I don't want recipes that have a long list of ingredients, ingredients that have to be purchased specially since they aren't kept on hand, or expensive ingredients. I want to prepare meals quickly with things that we always keep in stock. I am including some more complex recipes in a section at the end that are worth the effort for special occasions. If I am going to cook something more difficult, I make enough to eat for two or even three dinners so it is worth it! We don't require a lot of variety in our diet, and find the following typical meal plans work well for us and are also satisfying. Recipes for these are included in the 'Recipes' section.

The plans here might work for you, or they might not. The main thing is to include a variety of healthy food in your diet. Eat lots of vegetables of different kinds and colors. Eat a lot of salads, large salads. We make salads with all sorts of greens, carrots, avocados, sprouts, sunflower seeds, and whatever we happen to have. Eat a lot of beans, whole grains, nuts, and seeds. Eat some fruit. It isn't too difficult to get the nutrients you need.

Breakfast

We have two basic breakfast menus:

Oatmeal topped with fruit, sometimes with a scoop of homemade granola added in

Fruit smoothies with spelt toast spread with coconut oil and a sprinkle of salt.

Lunch

Tortilla wraps with pesto, leftover rice or quinoa, and salad vegetables
Tortilla wraps with humus and salad vegetables
Hummus with carrots and crackers
Tortilla wraps with leftover curry or stir fried vegetables
Black bean and vegetable burritos
Black beans and rice bowl
Mock tuna in a wrap
Leftover soup

Dinner

Soup and spelt bread
Quinoa salad
Vegan tortilla pizza
Blue corn black bean tacos
Pan sizzled tempeh with vegetables or salad
Miso soup with buckwheat soba noodles and vegetables
Vegetable or pumpkin curry with rice or quinoa
Cow peas with rice
Sweet potatoes or regular potatoes with a large salad

Special dishes to make for company or on special occasions

These take longer to make but are delicious!

Vegan mac & cheese (without cheese)
Vegan lasagna
Black bean & sweet potato enchiladas

Beverages

Coffee and tea -

Coffee can be made easily by pouring water through a Melitta type filter holder with a washable filter. We grind out coffee with a simple hand grinder, but you could also buy it ground although the flavor is better if you grind it yourself. If possible, it is best to purchase shade-grown, fair trade organic coffee. Shade-grown coffee is grown under the trees instead contributing to deforestation. It incorporates principles of natural ecology and provides habitat for the highest diversity of birds, native flora and fauna.

Tea is a wonderful option, and there are so many different interesting varieties and blends to experiment with. Try Kukicha twig tea or gunpowder green. We are buying it in bulk by subscription through Amazon since it is twice as expensive at our local stores and shipping is free even to Alaska. Tea bought in bulk is cheaper than tea bags, and we use a stainless steel mate spoon (bombilla) as a filter instead of a tea ball since it is easier.

You can save tons of money making your own coffee and tea instead of buying it by the cup, unless visiting coffee shops is a social thing for you. It is easy to keep coffee and tea hot in a simple thermos if you are away from home. Lots of people go through drive-through stands or visit coffee shops instead of making coffee at home and are tempted by all the special coffee drinks which are expensive and can be full of fat and sugar. One article I saw recently listed the calories of various specialty coffee drinks (not at all vegan!) at Starbucks and elsewhere and most were from 300-600 calories each! Yikes. If you meet someone for coffee or like the coffee shop atmosphere, consider bringing your own cup and taking it black.

Juice – From research I have done, I don't recommend drinking any fruit juice. Maybe if you make it yourself, but it is better to just eat the fruit and get the fiber since many brands add sugar and preservatives. V8 and commercial vegetable juices have salt and may be processed at high heat which lowers the nutrient content. Home juicers are good but it is one more appliance and many of them separate out the pulp which is good for you. If you want to make juice at home, I recommend using a blender which can be used for many other things.

Alcohol - Unless you have alcoholic tendencies, having beer and wine in moderation mainly with meals shouldn't be problematic and some studies show it has health benefits. They don't advise starting to drink for the benefits but it is encouraging for those of us who are seeking to rationalize our habit! Moderate is the key. I don't know about the credibility of the studies, but some claim moderate drinkers have a lower risk of developing type 2 diabetes, and that brain function declines less quickly. We stick with a glass or two of red wine with dinner which supposedly has antioxidants that may help prevent heart disease by increasing levels of "good" cholesterol which protects against artery damage. There is always the possibility that the studies were funded by the wine industry!

Wine is very expensive in Alaska, probably because it is heavy to transport. Besides the cost, we have no way to recycle glass and I don't like the plastic waste that comes from the boxed wine liner. Because of this, I have gotten into making my own wine from local fruit when I can get it, or from frozen grape juice. I like being in control of the chemicals added to the wine since commercially produced wine has various additives for killing bad bacteria, stabilizing, and clarifying the wine. Organic wine is hard to get and very expensive, and lots of pesticides are used to grow grapes. Making homemade wine isn't that difficult, but takes time and requires obtaining some basic equipment. There is too much information for me to go into here, but I will put some website links in the Reference section and include a very simple recipe that is made in a glass gallon jug at the end of the recipe section.

We get beer from a local brewery since we can use refillable growlers. It isn't organic, but it is excellent, supports a local business and is better than buying bottles we can't recycle.

Snacks

It is good to have some healthy snacks around that you can grab when you get hungry. Avoid mindless snacking or making a habit of snacking at a particular time of day, but if you are physically hungry it helps to eat something to take the edge off so you don't eat too much at meals. Sometimes we snack instead of a meal on particularly busy days. The following are things we usually have around:

Raw almonds – These are a wonderful snack. They are a good protein source and will fill you up. Raw nuts are better for you and not as addictive and temping as roasted/salted nuts. Any kind is good, but almonds seem easier to get in bulk at a good price. Walnuts are also really healthy, so we have them around also.

Apples and other fruit like oranges – Organic, naturally!

Dark chocolate chips – These work for me when I want something sweet because they are good, but not so good I want to eat lots of them. It is less expensive to buy them in bulk, and way cheaper than buying bars of chocolate in fancy packages.

Some studies have shown that dark chocolate is actually good for you since it is made from plants and contains flavonoids which act as antioxidants. Dark chocolate contains a large number of antioxidants (nearly 8 times the number found in strawberries) which have been investigated for the prevention of diseases such as cancer and heart disease. Studies show it lowers blood pressure, and it might even improve visual and cognitive functions – at least temporarily. Not that all this should be used as an excuse to eat lots of chocolate; it does have a lot of calories and it is best to keep it in small quantities. I love those study results though! Enjoy it while you can since they could decide the reverse is true tomorrow. I pay attention to the latest research on things, but don't hang my hat on it. Once again, use common sense and practice moderation with all things.

Popcorn – Air-popped, with a little melted coconut oil and nutritional yeast.

15

RECIPES

Writing 'organic' after all the ingredients in the following recipes seems repetitive, so assume that all ingredients should always be organic!

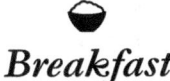

Breakfast

Oatmeal

Oatmeal is one of the healthiest and easiest breakfasts you can have. It is just as easy as boxed cereal, and is way better in many ways. We love steel cut oats which are really good, but take longer to cook and involves washing a pan. We buy rolled oats in bulk since it is much cheaper and saves packaging (don't chose instant oats since they are more processed). Quick oats are just cut thinner so they cook faster.

1 cup rolled oats per person

Simply put the rolled oats in a bowl, then add boiling water to cover them. Let them sit for a few minutes and you are ready to go. We sweeten it with molasses, add a sprinkle of cinnamon, some raisins or frozen blueberries, sometimes a scoop of homemade granola, and oat milk.

Oat Milk

Before giving up soy milk due to health concerns, I purchased a soy milk maker. Fortunately, this also makes other 'milk' as well. Almond milk is very good, but almonds are expensive and it was hard for us to find ways to use the pulp. I tried steel cut oats in the soy milk maker and it worked perfectly since they are very creamy. After straining out the milk, the remains are basically cooked cereal which can be then added to oatmeal or even put in the smoothie.

My electric soy milk maker is a cheaper model from Joyoung, but any of the others would probably work. You could also make oat milk by cooking the steel cut oats and then straining them, but this takes more time. I don't like having another electric appliance but this one definitely makes my life easier and is better than purchasing milk in aseptic containers which we have no means of recycling. Also, oat milk is very inexpensive to make, especially if you buy the steel cut oats in bulk.

Put ½ cup of uncooked steel cut oats into the soy milk maker, then add water to the fill line. Set the top with the motor in place, and plug it in. Push the 'make soy milk' button, and wait until it is finished processing. Strain the solids with the filter provided, and store the oat milk in the refrigerator. We have found that it keeps longer if we sterilize the jar used for storage with boiling water first.

Granola

6 cups oatmeal
1/2 cup sunflower seeds
1/4 cup flax seed
2 tsp cinnamon
2 tsp ginger
1/2 cup honey
1/3 cup melted coconut oil
1 cup raisins

Mix and bake at 325 degrees for 20 minutes, stirring occasionally.

Fruit Smoothies

My partner always makes the smoothies for our breakfast since he is better at it. I asked him for a recipe, and he basically said to mix a bunch of fruit with oat milk in the blender. Here are some approximate measurements to get you started.

Berry Smoothie

1 cup of frozen blueberries, blackberries, raspberries or a mix
4 large frozen strawberries
2 bananas
1Tb flax seeds

Add flax seeds to blender and blend to grind them, then add fruit and enough oat milk and water kefir to cover. Blend, adding more liquids if necessary. Any fruit could be used, and any type of milk (rice, almond, hemp, etc.).

Makes enough for two people.

Ginger Apple Smoothie

2 Tb grated fresh ginger
2 bananas
1 apple
1 pear (optional but delicious)
1 Tb flax seeds

Add flax seeds to blender and blend to grind them, then add fruit and enough oat milk and water kefir to cover. Blend, adding more liquids if necessary. Makes enough for two people.

Lunch

Pesto Wrap

spelt tortillas (recipe in 'Bread' section)
pesto sauce (recipes in 'Dinner' section)
hummus
rice or quinoa (leftovers)
grated carrot
cabbage or any green lettuce
avocado

Spread the tortilla with pesto sauce and fill with the above items or whatever sounds good to you!

Hummus Wrap

spelt tortillas
hummus (recipe to follow)
grated carrot
cabbage or any type of salad greens
sprouts
avocado

Spread the tortilla with Dijon mustard and fill with the above items.

Hummus

We make this at least once a week to eat with carrots or in tortilla wraps. I usually use dried garbanzos beans and make them in advance keeping extras in the freezer but you can also open a can. Just find an organic BPA free brand!

2 cups garbanzo beans or 1 can
1/4 cup tahini
1 tsp garlic powder (or one clove)
2 Tbs lemon juice
1 Tbs olive oil
1 tsp cumin
1/2 tsp season salt

Blend in a food processor until smooth.

Cooking garbanzo beans (Chickpeas):

To cook dry garbanzo beans on the stovetop, add three cups of water for each cup of dried garbanzo beans. Bring them to a boil, then reduce the heat and simmer, partially covering the pot. They generally take 2 hours depending on your heat source, and you might have to add more water so check them now and then. We cook them on a wood stove in the winter since it is always on.

Black Bean Burritos

Burritos are our most common lunch, and we have them several times a week. We usually cook a big pot of black beans on the woodstove or in the solar oven and use them throughout the week (see instructions below), but you could also open a BPA free can. You can put anything in your burrito, but this is what we usually put in ours.

　　spelt tortillas
　　black beans
　　leftover rice or quinoa
　　salsa
　　shredded cabbage
　　avocado

If your tortilla is too small, you can just stick the filling in and fold it over like a large taco.

Black Bean Bowl

　　black beans
　　brown rice or quinoa
　　shredded cabbage
　　salsa
　　avocado

Put cabbage in a large bowl, top with some rice, beans, salsa and some chunks of avocado.

Cooking black beans:

We eat a lot of black beans, and like them better than other varieties. I have a friend who swears by a pressure cooker, and it would be faster but we don't have one so these instructions are for the stove top method. The process is simple, and while they take a lot of time to cook it doesn't take much of your attention. We cook them on the woodstove top in the winter, and in the solar oven in the summer. We make a lot at a time since they keep for a week in the refrigerator and can be frozen.

Put your beans in a large pot, and sift through them to check for stones or discolored beans to discard. Cover them with water, and let them soak overnight. (Sometimes I leave out this step and haven't noticed any difference other than taking longer to cook, but supposedly it is better for gas issues.) Drain the beans, and add around 3 cups water for each cup of beans. I don't measure it out, and just cover them with plenty of water and drain it out at the end.

Bring them to a boil, then reduce it to a simmer and cook in a partially covered pot for until done. Depending on the temperature, this will take several hours or longer. Soaking the beans shortens the cooking time.

Mock Tuna

15 oz can garbanzo beans (chickpeas) drained, or 2 cups
   cooked dried garbanzo beans
2 tsp nutritional yeast
1 Tbs soy sauce
2 Tbs vegan mayo
1 Tbs minced onion

Blend in food processor. Good with crackers, or in a
wrap or sandwich with sprouts, shredded carrot, lettuce,
tomatoes, avocados, etc.

Bruschetta

*We only make this in the summer when we are growing fresh
tomatoes and basil, but it is something to look forward to.*

   2-3 large tomatoes, diced
   1/4 cup diced onion
   1/3 cup fresh basil
   1 clove garlic
   1 Tbs balsamic vinegar
   1 Tbs olive oil
   splash of soy sauce.

Mix and serve on toasted spelt bread.

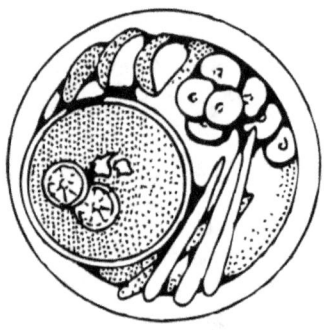

Dinner

Soups -

These are more appealing in winter, but wonderful all year round because they are inexpensive, full of nutritional ingredients and make enough for multiple meals. The extra can also be frozen for future fast food.

Split Pea Soup

2 cups dried split peas
1/4 cup barley
8 cups water
1 small onion, diced
1 clove garlic, diced
1 carrot, chopped
2 cubes vegetarian bouillon
splash of soy sauce
1/8 tsp cayenne
1 tsp cumin

Add barley and split peas to water, and simmer for 2 hours. Add everything else, and cook for another half hour or so.

Basic Vegetable Soup

4 cups water
1/2 cup lentils
1/4 cup barley
1 cube vegetable bouillon
1 potato
2 carrots
1 large can organic (non BPA lined) tomatoes or fresh
  equivalent
1 onion
1 cup mushrooms
3 cloves garlic
Seasonings to taste including pepper, seasoned salt, chili
  powder, and oregano.

Add lentil, barley and bouillon cube to water and bring to
a boil. Cut up potato and carrots and add them to the pot.
Add tomatoes. Sauté onion, mushrooms and garlic and add
to the pot. Season to taste, and cook another 30 minutes or
so until carrots are soft and lentils are done.

Curried Lentil Soup

5 cups water
1 cup lentils
1 small onion, diced
1 cup mushrooms, sliced
1 potato, diced
1 stalk celery, sliced
1 carrot, sliced
2 cloves garlic, minced
1 Tbs olive oil
2 tsp curry seasonings
1/2 tsp cumin
1/8 tsp cayenne
1/4 tsp ground ginger
1 Tbs. soy sauce
1/2 tsp seasoned salt
1 cube vegetarian bouillon

Sauté onions, mushrooms and garlic in oil in soup pot, then add water and lentils. Simmer for 20 minutes, then add other vegetables and seasonings and simmer for 1 hour.

Black Bean Soup

This is a crock pot recipe, but I gave ours away last time we moved so use the wood stove since it is cooked on low heat for hours. It has a lot of ingredients and takes a lot of time cooking, but it is so good and makes so much that it is worth it. I freeze half of it and it still gives us enough to eat for days. It is good when you are having a lot of company!

2 1/2 cups dry black beans
1 1/2 quarts water
1 carrot, chopped
1 large red onion, chopped
6 cloves garlic, minced
2 green bell peppers, chopped
2 jalapeno peppers, chopped
1/4 cup lentils
1 large can (28 oz) tomatoes or fresh equivalent
2 Tbs chili powder
2 tsp cumin
1/2 tsp oregano
1/2 tsp black pepper
3 Tbs red wine vinegar
1 Tbs. seasoned salt
1/2 cup brown rice

Soak beans overnight in a large pot, then drain. Combine soaked beans and water and cook on the woodstove or burner for 2 hours or until beans are getting soft (or in a crock pot on high for 5 hours). Stir in all other ingredients and cook for another hour (or in a crock pot on low for 2-3 hours). Cooking times may vary depending on temperature of method used.

Easy Pumpkin Soup

1/2 cup diced onion
2 cloves chopped garlic
1 16 oz can organic pumpkin
1 1/3 cup vegetarian bouillon
3 cups oat milk (or other 'milk')
1 Tbs curry powder
1 tsp oregano
Dash of soy sauce

Sauté onion, then add other ingredients and simmer for 15 minutes.

Quinoa Salad

cooked quinoa
salad greens or shredded cabbage
shredded carrots
sprouts
avocado

Put some cooked quinoa into a bowl, and put the salad ingredients above on top of it. Liberally sprinkle with seasoned rice wine vinegar and a splash of soy sauce or dressing (recipe below).

Lemon Vinaigrette
1 tsp sugar
1Tb lemon juice
1 Tb mustard
1/4 cup white wine vinegar
1 clove garlic
1/2 cup olive oil

Mix and store in the refrigerator.

Vegan Tortilla Pizza

This is one of my favorite recipes since it is so easy and reminds me of pizza.

spelt tortillas (recipe in 'Bread' section)
pesto sauce
walnuts
mushrooms
onions
broccoli, cut into small pieces

Put one tortilla for each person on a cookie sheet. Smear pesto on tortillas, and sprinkle with the above toppings. We use a lot of broccoli to make it more healthy!

Bake for 20 minutes at 400 degrees or until broccoli is soft and edges of tortilla are getting browned. It can also be cooked in a cast iron skillet on a woodstove or stove top.

Vegan Pesto Sauce

This is good on pasta, but we use it mainly for tortilla pizza sauce and in wraps with brown rice.

3 cups fresh basil
2/3 cup olive oil
5 cloves garlic
1/3 cup nutritional yeast
1/2 tsp salt
1/2 cup walnuts

Mix in blender (or food processor) until smooth. Freezes well.

Nasturtium Pesto

Nasturtiums grow easily, even in Alaska, and we use the leaves and flower in salads also.

4 cups packed nasturtium leaves
3 to 5 cloves of garlic
1 cups olive oil
1 cup walnuts

Mix in blender or food processor until smooth. Freezes well.

Blue Corn Black Bean Tacos

organic blue corn taco shells
black beans
avocados
sliced cabbage
salsa

We use the pre-made taco shells from Garden of Eatin' that are baked in the oven at 350 degrees for 5 minutes. Very easy! Stuff them with the ingredients listed above or whatever sounds good to you.

Miso Soup with Soba and Vegetables

Cook soba noodles according to package directions. We use buckwheat, and they come separated in serving size portions with paper bands. Drain them, and set them aside.

Stir fry a mix of vegetables like mushrooms, onions, and broccoli in a small amount of olive oil until done but still crisp. We usually cut up enough vegetables to fit in a cast iron skillet, and use up whatever we happen to have. Leftovers are appreciated the next day wrapped in spelt tortillas.

Put a tablespoon of miso paste (we use white) into each bowl and pour in hot water, mixing to dissolve. Add the cooked soba noodles and vegetables to the bowl.

Pumpkin Curry

8 cups water
1 cup dry lentils
1/2 cup dry brown rice
2 cups diced pumpkin
2 cloves chopped garlic
1/2 onion, chopped
1 1/2 cup sliced mushrooms
1 cube vegetable bouillon
2 Tbs curry powder
seasoned salt and pepper to taste

Add lentils and rice to water in a large soup pot and cook on the stove for 1/2 hour. Add pumpkin and cook another 20 minutes or until tender. Meanwhile, sauté garlic, onion and mushrooms and add to pot. Add bouillon cube, curry powder, and salt and pepper to taste. Serve with brown rice or quinoa.

Vegetable Curry

3 Tbs olive oil
1/8 tsp cayenne pepper (if you like it hot!)
2 Tbs (or more) curry powder
1 cup water
1 potato, cubed
Misc. chopped vegetables (cauliflower, broccoli, carrots, onions, etc.)

Heal oil, cayenne pepper, and curry in a cast iron pan, add potatoes and stir to mix. Add water and cover and simmer for 10 minutes. Add other vegetables and cook another 15 minutes. Add peas and cook until they are heated. Serve with brown rice or quinoa (instructions below). Leftovers are very good wrapped in a tortilla.

How to cook brown rice

I used to have a rice cooker, and it did make perfect rice but it wasn't necessary. We make it in a pan now, and it comes out just as good without yet another appliance to deal with.

Put 1 cup rice and 1 ½ cups water in a pot with a lid. Bring it to a boil uncovered, then put the lid on and reduce it to a simmer. Let is cook on low for 20 minutes, then turn off the heat and let it sit for another 10 minutes.

How to cook quinoa

Put 1 cup of quinoa in a pan and brown it, stirring it around to prevent burning. This gives it a good flavor. Add 2 cups of water and 1 vegetarian bouillon cube and simmer for 20 minutes with the lid on.

Cowpeas with Brown Rice

2 cups cowpeas or black-eyed peas
1 cup of diced onion
3 cloves garlic, minced
2 Tbs olive oil
4 cups veggie bouillon
1 cup brown rice
2 Tbs parsley
1 tsp oregano

Cover cowpeas with boiling water and let stand 20 minutes, then drain.

Sauté onion and garlic in olive oil and add cowpeas, rice, bouillon, parsley and oregano. Simmer until done. It is good with a Tbs of nutritional yeast to make it a little cheesy.

Dishes for company or special occasions

I love these recipes, but don't make them very often because they are more complicated and/or have more fat than I want on a daily basis. However, I am including them because they are delicious and good for special occasions or when company is coming to dinner.

Vegan Mac & Cheese (without cheese)

3 cups uncooked pasta (quinoa pasta is best)
1/4 cup coconut oil
1/4 cup spelt flour
1 3/4 cup oat milk
1 tsp season salt
1 Tbs soy sauce
1 tsp garlic powder or 1 clove minced
2 Tbs olive oil
1/2 cup nutritional yeast
2 cups bread crumbs (make toast and crumble it up)

Cook pasta according to package directions and set aside. In a ceramic cooking pot, melt oil and then mix in flour and cook until bubbly. Still in oat milk, soy sauce, garlic and stir until thick. Stir in oil and nutritional yeast, then add pasta. Top with bread crumbs and bake at 350 degrees for 20 minutes. Good with mushrooms or broccoli added. This tastes better than real macaroni & cheese to me!

Vegan Lasagna

This recipe is not difficult, but we don't eat a lot of pasta and tend to save it for when we are having guests for dinner since it can be made in advance then cooked before dinner, it makes a lot, and non-vegans even like it.

quinoa or rice lasagna noodles
1+ large jar spaghetti sauce
bunch of spinach or 1 chopped zucchini, sautéed
1/2 cup chopped walnuts
1 cup mushrooms, chopped
1/2 onion, chopped

Cook lasagna noodles according to package directions, drain and set aside (A little oil will keep them from sticking together). Sauté vegetables and set aside. Layer sauce, noodles, vegetables and walnuts in a large baking pan, repeat for 2nd layer. Bake uncovered at 350 degrees for 45 minutes.

Black Bean & Sweet Potato Enchiladas

Sauce: Add 4 cloves minced garlic and 4 Tbs minced onion to 2 Tbs olive oil and cook until translucent. Add 1 16 oz can tomato sauce, 1/2 cup salsa, 1/4 tsp salt, 1 tsp cumin, 1/4 tsp black pepper, 1 Tbs chili powder, and 1 tsp oregano. Simmer for 5-10 minutes.

Filling: Mix cooked black beans and cooked sweet potato. You can fill the enchiladas with anything that sounds good to you! Be creative. I don't have specific proportions since I usually wing it with whatever I have left over.

Dip corn tortillas in sauce, fill with black bean mixture, and roll them up. This is messy! Line up filled rolled tortillas in a baking pan. When the pan is full, pour sauce over the top and bake for 20 minutes at 350 degrees.

Bread

Spelt Tortillas

2 cups spelt flour
1/2 tsp salt
1/2 tsp baking powder
2 tsp oil
3/4 cup warm water

Mix all ingredients, cover and let rest for 10 minutes. Roll into 8 golf ball sized balls. Heat seasoned cast iron pan on high. Roll out one of the balls in a circle (a silicone mat with small silicone roller is best so it doesn't stick). I usually have to add flour to make them less sticky, and add flour to the mat and roller. Roll, turn a little, roll, turn a little until it is flat and round. Mine are not perfect, but it gets easier with practice. Make them as thin as you can but if they are too thin they will be hard to remove from the mat. When the pan is very hot, add the tortilla and cook a very short time on each side, a minute or less, until bubbles raise up on the surface. If the pan isn't hot enough you won't get the bubbles, but just cook it for a minutes and flip it over for 30 seconds or so on the other side. Leave them to cool on a rack, then they can be stored in the refrigerator for a week or in the freezer indefinitely.

Easy No-Knead Spelt Bread

2 1/2 cups warm water
1/4 tsp dried yeast
2 tsp salt
1 tsp honey
4 3/4 cup spelt flour

Mix all ingredient, cover with a plastic bag and let set overnight or for 12-15 hours. Punch down and fold over a few times, and let it sit 2-3 more hours until it has risen up again in the bowl. Sprinkle corn meal in the bottom of a dutch oven or ceramic pot and put it in the oven with the lid on. Heat oven to 500 degrees. When oven is hot, dump in the dough, put on the lid, and bake for 45 minutes. Remove the lid and bake another 10-15 minutes longer.

Quick Spelt Rolls

1 cup warm water
2 Tbs dry yeast
1/3 cup melted coconut oil
1/4 cup sugar
1 1/2 tsp salt
1 egg (or replacement listed at the end of chapter 2)
3 1/2 cup spelt flour

Mix water, oil, yeast and sugar and allow to rest for 15 minutes. Preheat oven to 400 degrees. Mix in salt, egg, and flour and briefly knead. Form into 12 balls, and place in greased pan. Let them rest 10 minutes, and bake for 15 minutes.

Desserts

Vegan Chocolate Mousse

This recipe is one I use if I need something for a special occasion, and it is so good that non-vegans won't realize it is made with tofu. We are generally avoiding tofu and soy products now, but this is a very occasional exception.

1/2 cup organic chocolate rice or hemp milk
1 small bag dark chocolate chips
12 oz package of silken tofu (it has to be silken tofu!)
1/2 cup almond liquor
1/4 tsp almond extract

Pour the chocolate milk into a small pot and warm slightly. Melt chocolate chips in a double boiler (pan over another pan with water in it). Stir occasionally until melted. Add chocolate, warmed milk, and tofu to blender and blend until smooth. Stir in liquor and extract then chill in a bowl for at least 1 1/2 hours. It will set as it cools.

Banana Sunday

banana, cut in slices and frozen
granola (see recipe under 'Breakfast')
peanut butter

Layer in a small bowl, and top with homemade magic shell.

Homemade Magic Shell

Melt 2 parts coconut oil with 3 parts dark chocolate (chips melt easier). Can store in a jar at room temperature. It might stay liquid depending on the temperature in your house, but is easy to warm up on a wood stove or in a pan of water on the stove. When poured on the frozen bananas, it will harden in a chocolate shell.

Chocolate Treats

1/2 cup coconut oil
1/3 cup sugar
3 Tbs cocoa powder
rolled oats
dried shredded coconut
peanut butter

Melt coconut oil and stir in sugar and cocoa powder. Add a big spoonful of peanut butter, and pour in 1/3 cup of coconut. Add oatmeal carefully until it is thicker but still flowing. Pour onto greased cookie sheet and stick in the freezer until firm. Break into chunks, and store in the freezer until ready to eat since it will get too soft at room temperature.

Beverages

Easy Grape Juice Wine

2 cans frozen grape juice (100 % juice)
2 1/2 cup sugar
2 tsp acid blend
1 tsp peptic enzyme
1 tsp yeast nutrient
1 campden tablet, crushed
1 packet wine making yeast

The wine making ingredients above can be found online in bulk, or at a wine-making store.

Campden tablets are a sulfide, and you could try leaving it out but one of the biggest problems with home wine making is having wild yeast and bacteria invade which can ruin the flavor. It is important to sterilize everything involved with boiling water or a product like Star San. I would rather not use any chemicals, but since I am new to this I am following instructions and erring on the side of caution. You will need to make sure the jug, counter, your hands, spoons, funnels, the cork and airlock, and anything you will be using has been sterilized prior to using it in wine making.

Boil 4 cups water with sugar and let cool. Add juice and other ingredients except for the yeast. Pour into a gallon jug, cover with a clean cloth napkin for 12 hours. Add the yeast and re-cover. After 5 days put a rubber stopper (#6 drilled with a hole to fit an airlock). The airlock should be half filled with sterilized water. When the activity has stopped and it is looking clear, pour it into another sterilized bottle (called racking) leaving the sediments behind and refit with the airlock. After 30 days, pour the wine off the sediment for a final time and bottle for drinking. You can just cap the jug and store it in the refrigerator which should stop any continued fermentation. If you store it at room temperature without adding stabilizing chemicals and the fermentation isn't totally finished, the pressure could build up and it might pop the top off.

There is a lot to learn with wine making so get a book or do internet research if you want to learn more. This recipe is a good way to get started since it is inexpensive and doesn't require much in the way of equipment. The drilled corks and airlocks are only a few dollars each, and the jugs can be found for free at a glass recycling center or you can save one from jugged wine or cider.

If you get further into wine making in larger batches, you might want 6 gallon carboys, a primary fermentation bucket, siphons, a hydrometer, a hand corker, etc. It is complicated at first, but gets easier and is well worth it if you enjoy drinking wine and want to save money and have more control over the additives. You can also purchase kits that have the grape juice from high end grapes in a sealed plastic bag, and various packets of chemicals to add with detailed directions. This will produce a better wine (Cabernet, Merlot, etc.) but I would leave out some of the chemical packets or research exactly what you will be adding and the consequences for leaving it out.

16

CONCLUSION

I sincerely hope this book inspires you to adopt or stick with a healthy vegan or 'mostly vegan' diet. Being healthy is the most important thing you can do; it effects how you feel, how you think and nearly every aspect of your life. How perfect that a mostly vegan diet is better for you and also better for the planet! These ideas are spreading, but not fast enough. I see huge supermarkets with shelves full of stuff that I don't think of as real food, and people filling their carts with slabs of meat, bags of chips, soda, and boxes of chemicals. It seems so clear that a whole food mostly vegan diet is superior, but lots of people aren't getting the message. I hope I can help spread the word, so feel free to share this book with anyone who could benefit from it!

I have included some links to good online sites for more information in the following reference section.

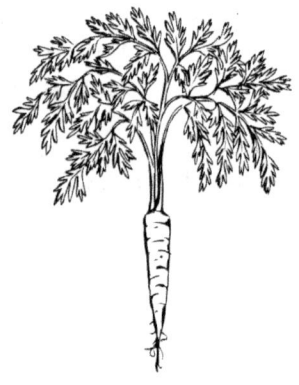

REFERENCES

For more information on topics covered in this book, follow the following links.

Cruelty to farm animals:
www.peta.org/issues/animals-used-for-food/factory-farming.aspx
www.green-blog.org/2010/07/22/the-cruel-life-inside-a-factory-farm/

Protein in the vegan diet:
www.vrg.org/nutrition/protein.htm

Egg replacers:
www.veganbaking.net/vegan-recipes/eggless-binders.html
www.veganwolf.com/vegan_cooking_substitutions.html

Why organic food is better:
www.organicconsumers.org/

Environmental problems associated with livestock:
www.veganoutreach.org/whyvegan/environment.html

Fermentation:
fermentationrecipes.com/ferment-airlock/889
www.fermentersclub.com/why-ferment/

Azure Standard:
www.azurestandard.com

United Natural Foods:
www.unfi.com/AboutUs.aspx

Food storage:
www.usaemergencysupply.com/information_center/
storage_life_of_foods.htm

BPA information:
en.wikipedia.org/wiki/Bisphenol_A
www.scientificamerican.com/article.cfm?id=plastic- not-
fantastic-with-bisphenol-a

Is chocolate good for you?
www.clinicalcorrelations.org/?p=4150
www.environmentalhealthnews.org/ehs/newscience/
dark-chocolate-may-improve-vision-memory

Is red wine good for you?
www.mayoclinic.org/diseases-conditions/heart-
disease/in-depth/red-wine/art-20048281

The soy controversy:
www.johnrobbins.info/blog/what-about-soy/

Giving up grains:
nourishedkitchen.com/against-the-grain-10-reasons-
to-give-up-grains/
articles.mercola.com/sites/articles/archive/2011/07/0
4/can-eating-this-common-grain-cause-psychiatric-
problems.aspx

Genetically Modified Food:
www.gmwatch.org/
www.huffingtonpost.com/2010/01/12/monsantos-gmo-
corn-linked_n_420365.html
ecowatch.com/2013/11/26/can-genetically-modified-
foods-trigger-gluten-sensitivity/

Fermentation:
articles.mercola.com/sites/articles/archive/2004/01/0
3/fermented-foods-part-two.aspx

Water Kefir:
www.yemoos.com/faqwahealth.html

Shade-grown coffee:
en.wikipedia.org/wiki/Shade-grown_coffee

Home winemaking:
winemaking.jackkeller.net/
www.eckraus.com/wine-making-steps/

"By eating meat we share the responsibility of climate change, the destruction of our forests, and the poisoning of our air and water. The simple act of becoming a vegetarian will make a difference in the health of our planet." - **Thich Nhat Hanh**

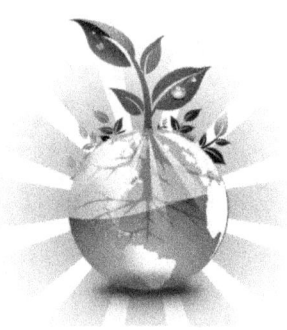

RECIPE INDEX

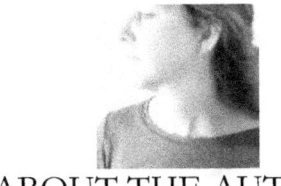

ABOUT THE AUTHOR

Michele Cornelius lives as sustainably as possible in a small town in Southeast Alaska with her pet duck, three cats, and her partner Gene. An ardent environmentalist, she enjoys being in wild places trying to capture the beauty of nature with photography.